MW01231814

Vagus Nerve

Mastery

A Self-Help Guide To Techniques And Daily
Exercises To Reduce Depression, Chronic
Illness, Anxiety, Digestive Problem

Harrison Thompson

Vagus Nerve Mastery

Vagus Nerve Mastery

Text Copyright©

Legal & Disclaimer

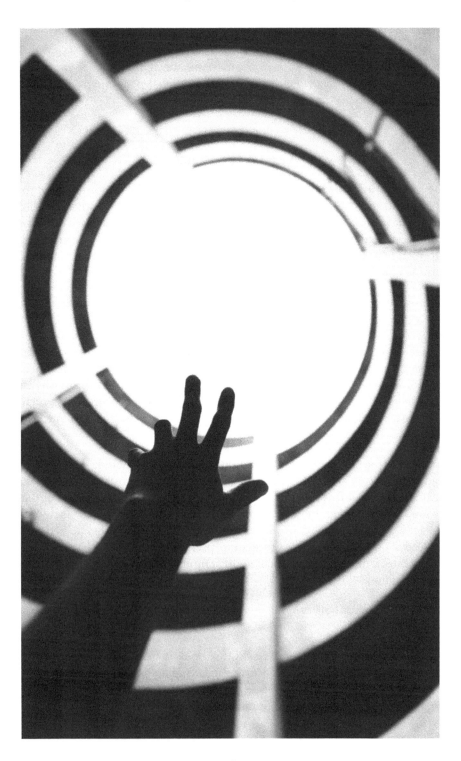

Table of Contents

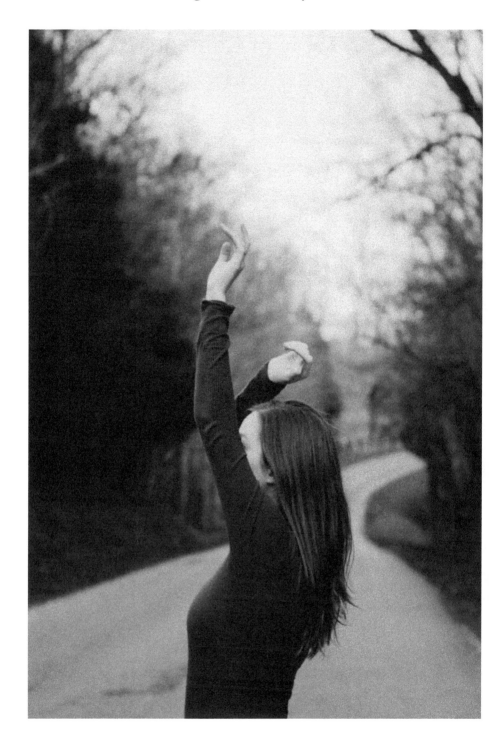

Introduction

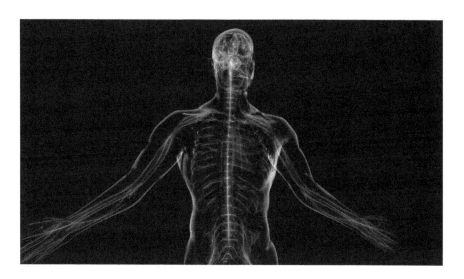

Our bodies are amazing. You don't even need to think in order to breathe, pump blood throughout your body, and process the food you ingest. Your body needs no conscious input from you to keep running and providing every cell in your body with the correct amount of nutrition, water, and oxygen to function perfectly. All this is made possible by your autonomic nervous system, which is responsible for all the unconscious functions of your body. Our brains are divided into sections, with the forebrain letting us think and consciously make decisions and do things. However, we don't need that section to survive. The brainstem manages that all on its own, without the need for any outside thought. You don't need to remember to breathe or keep your blood circulating, which is a good thing since most of us would probably forget sometimes.

The brainstem sits at the top of the spinal cord and is like the control center for all autonomic parts of the body. Each nucleus within the brainstem has a specific purpose and, when the connection between the brainstem and the rest of the body is damaged, it can wreak havoc on our bodies. Many people have discovered this firsthand when they suffer damage to their nervous system.

If you look at the brainstem as the computer that keeps the body running, your nervous system is like the cables that run to the various parts of the system. If one of those cables is damaged, it affects the entire system. Likewise, your body needs all those connections to function properly if you're going to feel great.

You have probably heard of the gut-brain connection. It postulates that a healthy gut results in a healthy brain. How could that possibly be? Well, you have connections throughout your body. The nervous system runs from your brain through your whole body, with the vagus nerve touching everything from your heart and lungs to the intestines and bladder. It's all connected and it isn't just the brain making things work throughout the body. What your body is going through is also a big part of your brain health. I liken it to a pond. If the pH is off or if one plant starts to overgrow, the entire system is wonky. It can be almost impossible to reset, because if you change the pH it changes everything. Just like that, if one part of your body is off, the rest of it will be altered, too, thanks to the nervous system.

Your nervous system can become damaged for a variety of reasons. Sometimes it's a disease that affects things. Sometimes it is a medication that is being used to treat something else. An accident or injury can also cause damage to the nervous system, and the results can be quite horrific and life-altering.

CHAPTER 1:

The Twelve Cranial Nerves

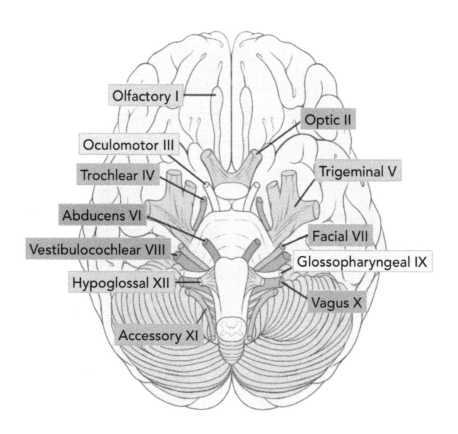

D id you know that the human body has 12 cranial nerves? Did you know that each "nerve" is actually comprised of two nerves, typically left and right nerve intertwined to make the "one" cranial nerve? And these nerves are the link between your body and the brain? Have you ever wondered how the brain and body "talk" to one another? It is all through these cranial nerves. Some of the nerves are responsible for sharing sensory information, like how something sounds or what it tastes like. This means these nerves need to have the sensory function to interpret the smell of something. But then there are other nerves that "talk" with the muscles and even some glands. These nerves are called "motor functions." And finally, while most have a single function, either sensory or muscle, others operate with both. The Vagus nerve is one such nerve.

To help you understand where a nerve is located, each cranial number is assigned a number represented in Roman numerals, for example, I is one, II is two, etc. The Vagus nerve is the tenth nerve and is called CNX, or Cranial Nerve Ten.

In Latin, the word "vagus" is defined as "wandering." When you understand a bit more about the makeup of this nerve, you will realize that this description is pretty accurate. The Vagus nerve is the longest in the human body, and it does a lot of traveling around and through it. Basically, it moves from the base of your skull to your lower torso.

Cranial Nerves

All of the cranial nerves are paired.

There are twelve (12) cranial nerves.

Each nerve is either a sensory nerve, a motor nerve, or both a sensory and a motor nerve.

All of the cranial nerves are part of the peripheral nervous system, except Cranial Nerve II

Cranial Nerves III through XII originate from the brainstem.

Some of the cranial nerves branch before their location of innervation is reached.

Cranial Nerve I

Name: Olfactory

Function: The special sense of smell, a SVA nerve – Special Visceral Afferent

Nucleus: Does not originate on the brainstem

Origin: Olfactory bulb

Exit from the Skull: Foramina in the cribriform plate

Component: SVA

Branches: Olfactory filaments

Sensory: Yes

Special Sense: Yes

Location: Nose

Cranial Nerve II

Name: Optic

Function: Sight

Nucleus: Lateral Geniculate Nucleus

Origin: Thalamus

Exit from the Skull: Optic foramen of the optic canal

Component: SSA

Branches: None

Sensory: Yes

Location (s): Retina of the eye

Special Sense: Yes

Cranial Nerve III

Name: Oculomotor

Functions: Control of many of the motor muscles of the eye and the constriction of the pupil as well as the accommodation of the eye

Nucleus: Oculomotor nucleus; GSE Nucleus

Nucleus: Edinger-Westphal nucleus; GVE Nucleus

Origin: Midbrain (mesencephalon region)

Exit from the Skull: Superior Orbital Fissure

Components: GSE and GVE

Branches:

Superior Branch (innervates the superior rectus and the levator palpebrae superioris)

Inferior Branch/Division – three branches

(1) Innervates the medial rectus

(2) Innervates the inferior rectus

(3) Innervates the inferior oblique and the ciliary ganglion

Somatic: Yes

Muscles Innervated: Muscles of the levator palpebrae superioris, superior rectus, medial rectus, inferior rectus, and inferior oblique muscles – these are extraocular muscles

Autonomic NS: Yes

Innervation: Parasympathetic via the Edinger-Westphal nucleus

Motor: Yes

Location: Most of the muscles of the eye

Cranial Nerve IV

Name: Trochlear

Function: Manages the superior oblique muscle of the eye, it rotates the eyeball

Nucleus: Trochlear nucleus

Origin: Midbrain

Exit from the Skull: Superior Orbital Fissure

Component: GSE

Branches: None

Somatic NS: Yes

Muscles Innervated: Superior oblique

Motor: Yes

Location: Superior oblique muscle

Cranial Nerve V

Name: Trigeminal

Functions: Sensory from the face and the muscles of mastication

Nucleus: Trigeminal nuclei

Origin: Pons

Exit from the Skull: Superior orbital fissure – V1; GSA component

Exit from the Skull: Foramen rotundum – V2; GSA component

Exit from the Skull: Foramen ovale – V3; SVE component, GSA component

Components: GSA - Sensory from the face and SVE - motor muscles of mastication

Branches: V1 – the ophthalmic nerve; V2 – the maxillary nerve; and V3 – the mandibular nerve

Somatic NS: Yes

Locations: V1 receives sensory information from the upper portion of the face. V2 receives sensory information from the middle region of the face. V3 supplies sensory information from the lower portion of the face.

Sensory: Yes

Motor: Yes

Special Sense: Yes

Other: There are three main branches of the Trigeminal nerve. They are designated by the following abbreviations: V1 (ophthalmic), V2 (maxillary), and V3 (mandibular). The trigeminal nerve has both sensory and motor components. V1 and V2 contain only sensory information. The V3 nerve is designated in the special visceral efferent (SVE) functional group.

Cranial Nerve VI

Name: Abducens

Function: Abducts the eye

Nucleus: Abducens nucleus

Origin: Pons, junction with the medulla

Exit from the Skull: Superior orbital fissure

Component: GSE

Branches: None

Somatic NS: Yes

Muscles Innervated: Lateral rectus muscle

Motor: Yes

Location (s): Lateral rectus Muscle

Cranial Nerve VII

Name: Facial

Functions: Muscles of facial expression, taste and gland stimulation (allows some people to wiggle their ear)

Nucleus: Facial motor nucleus - SVE

Nucleus: Superior salivatory nucleus – GVE

Nucleus: Geniculate ganglion - GSA, SVA, GVA

Origin: Junction of the pons and the medulla

Exit from the skull: Stylomastoid foramen

Components: GSA, GVA, SVA, GVE, and SVE

Branches: Cranial Nerve VII has intracranial and extracranial branches.

Intracranial: The greater petrosal nerve; nerve to stapedius; and the chorda timpani

Extracranial: The posterior auricular; the posterior branch of the digastric muscle as well as the stylohyoid muscle; and the five facial branches as follows: temporal; zygomatic; buccal; marginal mandibular; cervical

Somatic NS: Yes

Muscles Innervated: Posterior auricular

Autonomic NS: Yes

Innervation: General visceral efferent (GVE) to the submandibular, lacrimal, and sublingual glands as well as the mucosa of the nasal cavity.

Sensory: Yes

Location (s): Sensation from the posterior ear (GSA) and sensation from the soft palate and nasal cavity (GVA), anterior 2/3 of tongue, most of the muscles of the face

Motor: Yes

Special Sense: Yes

Cranial Nerve VIII

Name: Vestibulocochlear

Functions: Hearing and Balance: the vestibulocochlear nerve mediates the sensation of sound, rotation, and gravity, which is essential for balance and movement. The vestibular branch carries impulses for equilibrium while the cochlear branch carries impulses for hearing

Nucleus: Spiral ganglia - hearing

Nucleus: Vestibular ganglion - balance

Origin: Lateral side of the medulla and the lateral end of the trapezoid body of the pons.

Exit from the Skull: Interior Auditory Canal

Component: SSA

Branches: Two branches - Cochlear nerve; vestibular nerve

Sensory: Yes

Location: Ear

Special Sense: Yes

Other: Cranial nerve VIII has two main components and functions. It functions in both the special senses of hearing and balance (equilibrium). There are two main branches of this nerve – the vestibular nerve and the cochlear nerve. The vestibular nerve functions in balance, the cochlear nerve functions in hearing. Hearing and balance are both special senses, and both of these nerve branches contain sensory neurons.

Cranial Nerve IX

Name: Glossopharyngeal

Functions: Multiple Functions: General Somatic Afferent (GSA) sensory information from the tympanic membrane, upper pharynx and the posterior one third of the tongue, GVE neurons – parasympathetic innervation that causes salivation, SVE innervation - Brachialmotor function, taste, General Visceral

Afferent (GVA) sensory information from the carotid sinus and the carotid body

Nucleus: Solitary nucleus – SVA, GVA

Nucleus: Nucleus ambiguus

Nucleus: Inferior salvatory nucleus - GVE

Nucleus: Spinal nucleus of the trigeminal nerve

Nucleus: Lateral nucleus of the vagal trigone

Origin: Upper medulla

Exit from the Skull: Jugular Foramen

Components: GVA, GVE, SVE, GSA, SVA

Branches: The tympanic nerve; the stylopharyngeal branch, tonsillar branches, nerve to carotid sinus, branches to the posterior tongue, lingual branch, and a communicating branch to the vagus and it contributes to the pharyngeal plexus.

Somatic NS: Yes

Innervation: Tympanic membrane, upper pharynx and the posterior one third of the tongue

Autonomic NS: Yes

Innervation: General Visceral Efferent (GVE) (neurons from the parotid gland via the Otic Ganglia)

Sensory: Yes

Motor: Yes

Special Sense: Yes

Location: This nerve provides the sensation of taste to the posterior one-third of the tongue, as well as the circumvallate papillae, Special Visceral Efferent (SVE) nerves to the Stylopharyngeal muscle, carotid sinus and the carotid body

Other: With cranial nerve X, the glossopharyngeal, is involved in the gag reflex.

Cranial Nerve X

Name: Vagus

Functions: Multiple Functions: parasympathetic innervation, sensory information, taste to the epiglottis of the tongue, parasympathetic innervation to the glands of the mucous membranes of the pharynx, larynx, organs in the neck, thorax, and abdomen

Nucleus: Dorsal nucleus of the vagus nerve – parasympathetic innervation to the intestines and viscera - GVE

Nucleus: Nucleus ambiguus – to the brachial efferent neurons and the parasympathetic neurons to the heart

Nucleus: Solitary nucleus – afferent from taste and afferent from the viscera

Nucleus: Spinal trigeminal nucleus

Origin: Lateral side of the medulla

Exit from the Skull: Jugular Foramen

Components: GVE, SVE, SVA, GSA, GVA – general sensory innervation from the thorax and abdominal viscera

Branches: The auricular nerve; pharyngeal nerve; superior laryngeal nerve; superior cervical cardiac of vagus; inferior cervical cardiac; recurrent laryngeal nerve, branches of the pulmonary plexus; branches of the esophageal plexus; anterior vagal trunk; posterior vagal trunk

Somatic NS: Yes

Innervation: External auditory meatus and the tympanic membrane, pharynx, larynx, organs of the neck, thorax and abdomen

Autonomic NS: Yes

Sensory: Yes

Locations: The tongue, muscle of the pharynx and the larynx, sensation from the external auditory meatus and tympanic membrane, general somatic afferent (GSA), GVA – from the thoracic and abdominal visceral including the aortic arch and aortic body

Motor: Yes

Special Sense: Yes

Other: With cranial nerve IX, the vagus, is involved in the gag reflex.

Cranial Nerve XI

Name: Spinal Accessory

Function: Motor function of the sternocleidomastoid and the trapezius

Nucleus: Spinal accessory

Origin: Cranium and upper spinal cord

Exit from the Skull: Jugular foramen

Component: SVE

Branches: None

Motor: Yes

Location: Sternocleidomastoid and the trapezius

Special Sense: Yes

Other: Cranial nerve XI is the only cranial nerve that originates in the spinal cord, it then ascends into the cranial space, later it exits the cranium through the jugular foramen

Cranial Nerve XII

Name: Hypoglossal

Functions: Motor muscles of the tongue; speech, the formation of food bolus – manipulating food in the mouth, swallowing

Nucleus: Hypoglossal nucleus

Origin: Medulla oblongata

Exit from Skull: Hypoglossal Canal

Component: GSE

Branches: None

Somatic NS: Yes

Muscles Innervated: Genioglossus, geniohyoid, hyoglossus, styloglossus, thyrohyoid

Motor: Yes

Location: Muscles of the tongue

Main Cranial Nerves Dysfunctions and Social Engagement

Currently, the psychological state of modern humanity is not positive. There is a consistent rise in anxiety, depression, and stress. And even more troubling is the psychological distress is affecting younger ages, including teenagers and even young children. Many factors contribute to this increase in mental and emotional destabilization; however, it can probably be related to the confusion about the truth of human condition, misprescribed medication for emotional states, increases in isolation and social loneliness levels, constantly and quickly changing society, and faced-paced lifestyles.

Adaptive and Maladaptive

Now that you have the foundational understanding of how your consciousness works, you are ready to explore the process of experiencing emotions. This is why some people "process" or "handle" their emotions one way instead of another. Some processing is productive and "good" for you, while there are other "coping strategies" for emotions that are not as helpful. These "other" strategies are called "maladaptive." In the example above regarding an adult's response to an emotional child, there can sometimes be discord between public emotional display or the private self and one's core feelings. If you judge yourself or others negatively for experiencing a "negative" emotion, this will probably create conflict. This conflict can exist intrapsychically, or within yourself, or interpersonally, or another person judging you.

Common Symptoms of a Malfunctioning Vagus Nerve

Some may say that the Vagus nerve is the most important cranial nerve in your body. Others may disagree that it is the most important, but almost everyone can agree that it is vital to your well-being. Your optimal health, your most healthy life, requires a properly functioning Vagus nerve. The nerve does extend through some of your most vital organs and systems, such as your brain, esophagus, heart, lungs, and digestive tract. It also has the widest distribution of sensory and motor nerves in the body. It is responsible for the things in your body that you do not need to think about, like digestion and heart rate. It is pretty important.

But what happens when things go wrong? That is when you get disorders and malfunctions. Your Vagus nerve can be underactive or overactive. An overactive Vagus nerve can lead to increased stress and anxiety. An underactive Vagus nerve can lead to gastroparesis, which then can lead to diabetes. Before things get too "bad," you will typically get some warning signs. These symptoms are messages that there is either a disorder or damage to your Vagus nerve. Chances are, if you notice these symptoms, especially early on, you can do something about it. And most likely the best thing for you to do is to stimulate your Vagus nerve. As mentioned above, your Vagus nerve can be overstimulated or under-stimulated. This means your symptoms can be classified under one "type" of the problem or another. Sometimes the symptoms will overlap, but for the most part, you can identify the underlying issue for your Vagus nerve and take steps to correct it. One of the most common issues with Vagus nerve malfunctions is that it appears to be IBS or Irritable Bowel Syndrome. The symptoms can be similar. Moreover, physicians have a hard time diagnosing the condition in the Vagus nerve, primarily because the conditions do not usually show up in routine testing unless things have become really bad.

Vagus Nerve Damage – Common Symptoms

Before going any further regarding the malfunction, it is important to recognize the most common symptoms:

• Pain

• Organ Dysfunction

• Muscle Cramps

• Difficulty Swallowing

• Fainting

• Peptic Ulcer

• Gastroparesis

Pain and the Vagus Nerve

The common symptom for a malfunctioning Vagus nerve is a pain. But to know that the pain you are feeling is related to your Vagus nerve requires you to identify how the pain manifested in your body, where it is happening, and what the pain is trying to tell you. You need to understand the pain you are experiencing. Vagus nerve pain is caused by pressure, trauma, or injury that is mechanical. This leads to inflammation and swelling. Most of the time the pain you are experiencing is from a pinched nerve. The nerve leaves the skull through small foramina. This pain is vague and relatively flat. It is not constant or sharp. It will not feel like someone is stabbing you or lasting for stretches of time.

Organ Dysfunction and the Vagus Nerve

This nerve is long. Like mentioned earlier, it goes through several different important organs. When there is damage to the nerve, the organs fail to get the signal from the brain and the brain fails to get the information it needs from the organs. If there is damage to the nerve fibers the symptoms you will feel will be localized and represent symptoms of organ dysfunction. This does not result in your organs not working all of a sudden but it does mean that some of the functions will be less or absent.

Difficulty Swallowing and the Vagus Nerve

As mentioned earlier, the Vagus nerve is responsible for your esophagus and vocal chord function; however, when there is a problem with the Vagus nerve, there can be a problem. One of those problems includes your gag reflex. Just like a patient who has suffered from a stroke or head trauma and has trouble swallowing now, when a patient has damage to their Vagus nerve, they can experience trouble swallowing. If you are having trouble swallowing and also have a change in your gag reflex, you likely have a problem with your Vagus nerve. The major worry with this is the increased risk of choking. The start is just general challenges with swallowing and compounds from there.

Fainting and the Vagus Nerve

Fainting is a serious side effect of the Vagus nerve malfunction. This is a symptom of an overstimulated and overactive Vagus nerve. When you get this sudden fainting symptom you can collapse. The action of fainting is not necessarily dangerous by itself, but then, you collapse because of it, you increase the risk of physical injury.

Peptic ulcer and the Vagus Nerve

If there is damage to the Vagus nerve, another symptom and condition of this damage can be the development of a peptic ulcer.

The damage of the nerve may be stopping the beneficial mechanisms of control, which are in charge of the secretion of gastric acid. When this impairment occurs you may end secreting more peptic acid than normal. This then results in various conditions and diseases related to the gastrointestinal tract, like ulceration, gastroesophageal reflux disease, and dyspepsia.

Gastroparesis and the Vagus Nerve

This condition has been mentioned a couple of times already and now deserves its listing of symptoms for a dysfunction of the Vagus nerve. This is caused when your Vagus nerve is underactive. When this happens there is a negative impact on the blood supply to your stomach after you ingest food. When this happens, it is common to feel painful cramping or a stabbing sensation in your abdomen. You may also experience painful spasms. This painful reaction can then lead to heartburn, nausea, and unintended weight loss. It will also likely impact your typical intake of food.

More on Gastroparesis

This is a serious condition that impacts typical and spontaneous stomach muscle movement. In more healthy humans, the contractions in your stomach are strong propulsion for your food to move into your digestive tract. But if you suffer from gastroparesis, the movement in your stomach muscles is slower or not functioning at all. This stops your stomach from emptying the contents like it is supposed to.

The Spinal Nerves

The central nervous system is created from the brain and therefore the funiculus. Whereas the peripheral nervous system is actually made up of an associate interconnection of nerve fibers with the central nervous system, it functions commonly during a well-outlined pattern. The interconnections may be the advanced part. The body functions in coordinated motions. When sensing changes it adjusts itself to the correct surroundings. The system may well be a very advanced section of an associate animal that coordinates its actions and sensory data by sending signals to and from completely different components of its body. The system detects environmental changes that impact the body and so works with the system to resort to such events.

The peripheral nervous system principally consists of nerves. It is created from the enteric and involuntary nervous system. Bodily nerves mediate voluntary movement. The involuntary system is divided into some basic parts: the sympathetic and the parasympathetic nervous systems.

The sympathetic system is activated in cases of emergencies to mobilize energy whereas the parasympathetic system is activated once organisms unit in an exceedingly, in a very relaxed state. The enteric system functions to control the system. Every involuntary and enteric nervous system operate involuntarily.

Nerves that exit from the bone unit are referred to as cranial nerves. Whereas those exiting from the funiculus unit are referred to as spinal nerves. At the very cheap level that hinges on the cellular, a special quite cell that is termed the somatic cell. Neurons are capable of causing signals to completely different cells, and these signals travel so much through axons that are square measure typically to blame for secreting neurochemicals at junctions known as synapses. Most times once a cell receives any signal from the cell, responses may be redoubled or minimized.

Cnidarians (which embrace anemones, hydras, corals and jellyfish) accommodates a diffuse nerve web. All different animal species, except a couple of kinds of a worm, have a system containing a brain, a central twine (or 2 cords running in parallel), and nerves divergent from the brain and central twine. The scale of the system ranges from a couple of hundred cells within the simplest worms to around three hundred billion cells in African elephants.

CHAPTER 2:

The Polyvagal Theory

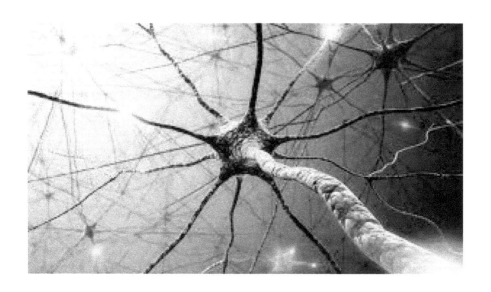

D evelopmental outcomes, physiology, and social engagement are explored in the neurobiological theory, the Polyvagal Theory. It is a complicated theory that can get convoluted. The design of this chapter is to help break down the theory into a three-part introduction. To begin, you need to know more about stress and the physiology of it as well as various responses to stress that occur in your body.

Your Nervous System

There are two primary nervous systems in your body, your peripheral nervous system, or PNS, and your central nervous system, or CNS. The CNS is your spinal cord and brain. It controls thoughts. The PNS is all the other nerves as well as ganglia. These regulate the limbs, organs, and muscles. The PNS is the autonomic nervous system, or ANS, and the somatic nervous system. Both are responsible for involuntary and voluntary functioning. For example, talking, seeing, smelling, as well as digesting and breathing. Then the ANS is broken down into the parasympathetic and sympathetic nervous system. This is the "fight, flight, or freeze" impulse and "rest and digest." When you relax and let yourself be calm, you signal your parasympathetic nervous system to "rest and digest." But if you become afraid or stressed, you have a physiological response. This is your sympathetic nervous system, or your "fight, flight, or freeze" response. Your body is responding to mobilize and handle the "threat." Your heart beats faster, pupils dilate, saliva production increases, and your blood sugar increases.

When you are threatened or afraid, the model is fairly straightforward. Your body responds to a problem. But there are a lot of things that are still unanswered or are a variable. For instance, is there always either a parasympathetic response or a sympathetic response or can you operate without one of those responses? How does the body respond when the body is chronically stressed? Why does a body trigger the "fight, flight, or freeze" response when you see something dramatic on television when you know it is not real or is not life-threatening. Are emotions necessary for these responses?

Humans are "hard-wired" to be social and in groups. This means that social engagement is entangled with how you respond physiologically. This has led to humans coping with stressors that are urgent and impactful on the immediate self but also stressors that are social in nature, too. This theory, the Polyvagal Theory, attempts to stitch together factors of these responses on a social, physiological, and evolutionary platform. But before getting into these factors, it is good to have a review of the Vagus nerve and how it deals with the regulation of your stress levels.

The Healing Power of the Polyvagal Theory

Part of the Polyvagal Theory explored earlier in this book, is what some people call the "social nerve system." Dr. Stephen Porges developed this concept, going on to describe how the social nerve system is a portion of the brain where the eyes, voice, and facial expressions are influenced and are used to influence others. The reason babies are so often used as examples for this theory is that human babies are born helpless. They need protection and support as they continue to develop. Because they cannot walk or talk, the infant human body adapted with skills designed to activate the social nerve system in the adult. While modern science may still only recognize or discuss two nervous systems, the sympathetic and parasympathetic, there is a third that needs to be injected into the system that offers an explanation to the gaps that still exist when it is just the two polarities. Each one of the systems is designed to deal with stress in a different manner. For example, think of an infant who shifts its body to face toward their parent, and uses their eyes and facial gestures to signal his or her parents. If this fails and no one acknowledges the message she or he is trying to send, the parasympathetic nervous system is activated and the infant begins to get angry and cry. And if this message still goes unanswered, the infant can then "play dead," becoming quiet and still. As the infant learns how the different responses and strategies work, the more it becomes ingrained in their subconscious and used as they grow into an adult.

This third system, the social nervous system, makes sense. The entire body and mind, including your nervous system, seeks balance inside and out. It wants to not only be harmonious in its internal functioning, but it also wants to feel harmonious with its surroundings. This is why, when your life is stressful and "stormy," you probably have a natural tendency or inclination to reach out to someone to find empathy. You want or even need to share with others because it is important for your survival to know that you are not alone and that what you are going through is not just a "you" thing or something that sets you apart from the rest. With this information now in your "tool belt," you may feel like a fog has dissipated and you can finally see yourself and others more clearly now. Now that you know the social nervous system and the three systems and responses, you can recognize the stage a person is in. Not only does this help you, but it helps you see how other people are doing around you. Are they shutting down and "playing dead" because you or others have failed to acknowledge their needs? Or are they screaming for attention? Can you try and catch them when they are engaging their social nervous system and displaying the Polyvagal Theory in their facial expressions?

Your body and brain send out various energetic frequencies. Think about brain waves. These are like sound waves and are measurable frequencies. Researchers, such as Dr. Joe Dispenza, identified that infant brain waves are primal and connected to the development of the subconscious. During this time the subconscious is being developed and finalized with the important survival needs. It is developing a strategy to help you survive as you grow and later in life. When the infant reaches childhood, the brain waves and frequencies shift. They become more creative. Imagination and creative play, like turning an everyday object into a monster, dinosaur or horse. It is also why monsters live under the bed, etc.

These frequencies do not leave you when you become an adult, but often they become only active right before and just as you fall asleep. It is also common just when you wake up or when you are deep in meditation. These connections are very close to the subconscious. In these states, you have the ability to change the pattern of your neurology and "reprogram" what you learned as an infant and young child about survival among other things.

When you turn ten your brainwaves and energetic frequencies change again. Now they are more "mature" and follow a more rational approach. This change continues throughout adulthood. At this point the brain can identify the difference between different things, like the everyday object is not really a dinosaur and the shadow is just a shadow, not a monster. In addition, it provides the ability to rationalize emotions and situations. For example, you can find a rational reason why you should not deal with your emotions. But while you may convince your mind not to deal with it, eventually it will come out, and your body will respond in ways you cannot or do not want to control. You rationalize yourself into illness. At this point, you have learned about the various stages of brain and energy waves, as well as the three nervous systems; social, sympathetic, and parasympathetic.

You have also been introduced to the idea that the way adults respond to stressful situations, in particular, is due to the strategies they found which worked best for them when they were children. From a neuroscience point of view, this information is transformational. This information shows that the immune system, endocrine, and nervous system are all connected and working together inside you.

The concept is basic; if you are socially unable to cope with your stress, the body then begins to "fight, flight, or freeze." This physiological state is not a place you want or should stay in long. If you do not cope with this threat or stress quickly, your body and mind start to fade. How you choose to interact with others includes the degree of interaction as well as the manner of contact. This determines the majority of your health. To find this balance and harmony, you need to do more than just meditate for 15 minutes every day by yourself or do a 30-minute relaxation yoga video by yourself. This is why the third system, the social nervous system, regulated largely by the Vagus nerve, supports your need to connect. Think about the importance of going to church on a Saturday or Sunday. You can pray at home but it is important to be together with others that support your view on spirituality. It is also why going to a fitness class is a far different outcome, especially on your happiness, than doing a program at the house by yourself. This means it is not about the actions physically, but about the connection socially. Studies at this stage people's brain waves become calmer and more peaceful. And all of this knowledge then leads to a powerful change agent you can use in your future.

Stress and the Sympathetic Nervous System

The Vagus Nerve and Stress Regulation

This "wandering" nerve that stretches from your brainstem to your colon has about 80% of its nerve fibers working in one capacity; to send information from the organs in your body to your brain. This type of nerve fiber is called afferent fibers. This information alerts your brain about what your organs are doing, like if your heart is beating at a normal rate or faster, or if you are having trouble with digestion or if it is functioning properly, or if your pupils are dilated or not. The other almost 20% of the nerves are efferent, or "highways" for the brain to tell your organs to do different things. This will be discussed in more detail later in this chapter. The Vagus nerve has a very important role in the regulation of the body. Its primary job is to make sure everything is balanced with one another. This is called "homeostasis." This relates to things like body temperature, chemistry in your body, activation, etc. And what is even more amazing is that the homeostasis of an organ can be different depending on the context of the situation, meaning the Vagus nerve interprets the context in which you are living and works with the organs to respond evenly to that.

To help illustrate this point, think about what happens to your body when the weather is hot. Blood takes a longer route, moving around your body to spread out the heat, but when the temperatures drop and it is cold outside, your blood changes its average course, favoring your major organs over your extremities. Even the arteries in your legs and arms constrict in the cold to minimize the amount of blood flowing into them so it can keep your organs warm. It may be frustrating to suffer from cold fingers and toes but it is your body's way of keeping your body temperature balanced for your internal organs. Next time you experience this, take a moment to thank your Vagus nerve for doing its job and put on warmer clothing without complaint!

Social stressors can also change the equilibrium of your body. The average heart beats between 60 and 80 times every minute when it is relaxed. But if a bear chases you, or you are running a marathon, your heart should pump faster to spread more oxygen out. In both scenarios, the primary goal for your body is to go a further distance. The extra blood and oxygen are being utilized to help you reach that goal. But when you feel nervous or see something disturbing on television your heart also picks up the pace. Think about before the first day of work, the morning of a big exam, preparing to walk on stage for a large presentation, etc. All of these situations typically lead to a faster heart rate. These situations may seem strange to have more blood and oxygen racing around your body. You are not preparing your body to fight or run, but your body is responding like it is. It is acting the same as if a bear all of a sudden rounded the corner to maul you, instead of just saying hello to a nice, attractive, special person. These "other" situations are explained in the Polyvagal Theory to define why this happens.

"Polyvagal" is used to describe the branches of the Vagus nerve. There are two types; unmyelinated and myelinated. A Myelin Sheath is a substance primarily made of fat that lines various nerves. It is meant to aid signals so they are sent to the brain faster and more accurately. If a nerve does not have a myelin sheath, it is called unmyelinated and it functions more primitively. The messaging from these nerves is not as fast or organized. To help you visualize the difference between the two, think about cars traveling on a well-designed and maintained road with strategic stoplights and a speed limit sign. The road is designed to help passengers travel quickly and easily but is controlled to maintain the safety of all the passengers on it. This is a "myelinated" road. Now visualize a dirt road winding around backcountry with no regulations in place and no clear direction. The journey is more troublesome and dangerous for all the travels passing along it. In addition, with the bumps and the uneven surface, it is harder to travel quickly. This is an "unmyelinated" road.

The branches of the Vagus nerve and all the nerves in the body are meant to keep your body balanced and functioning well. This is accomplished with three neural control stages. These three stages are operating in the unmyelinated branch of the Vagus nerve, the sympathetic adrenal system, and the myelinated branch of the Vagus nerve. There are different times for operation and a variety of effects each stage produces in and on the body when it is activated.

The unmyelinated branch of the Vagus nerve can be considered the least evolved of all the stages. This is because it is a more primitive evolution of communication in the body, and it is seen in primitive vertebrates, amphibians, and various reptiles as well. As animals evolved, coping skills for stress evolved to be more effective on a physiological level.

Below is a table that outlines the different stages, from least evolved to the most, along with the behavioral functions each stage deals with.

Stage Number	Component Utilized	Behavior and Function	"Lower Motor Neurons"
3	Myelinated branch of the Vagus nerve	Inhibits sympathetic-adrenal influences, related to calming and social-soothing as well as social communication	Nucleus ambiguus
2	Sympathetic-adrenal System	Actively avoiding, mobilization	Spinal cord
1	Unmyelinated branch of the Vagus nerve	Passive avoidance, feigning death, immobilized	Dorsal motor nucleus of the Vagus nerve

There is a fine balance struck between inhibition and excitation. This means that when one is active, the others are inactive. When one is "on," the others are "off." When you are facing common, everyday stress, like a deadline at work of having a fight with your partner or having a lot of homework to do, your body tends to suppress two states, favoring the reliance on your more evolved step, the myelinated Vagus nerve. But when stress becomes too great, your body drops to the next stage, which is more primitive. And then further, if compounded.

Unmyelinated Vagus Nerve Introduction

This is the most primitive response to your environment. This is about immobilization or even fainting, which is common in humans at this stage. Animals feign death when activating their unmyelinated Vagus nerve. The main goal of this response is to conserve your resources. This is especially seen in your heart rate. Bradycardia, or a low, maintained heart rate, is often the outcome of this state. Some animals and most reptiles use this to mimic death, but humans need more oxygen than these animals. In fact, all mammals would suffer severe damage if they feigned death in this manner. To see examples of this, research sharks when they go into the "shark trance" or snakes when they experience tonic immobility. It is clear that this response is not always very effective, which is most likely why humans have evolved to not use this response often. You probably will not be in this stage on a regular basis, certainly not during your day-to-day activities. This stage is activated only when there is extreme stress.

If someone experiences this stress and response chronically, they suffer from an illness called "vasovagal syncope." These people faint when they are triggered in different situations or experience extreme stress. Emotional triggers are also known to cause this response for people with this diagnosis, such as seeing blood. It can also occur from standing too long. It is unknown what causes this disorder but some experiments conducted on animals suggest it is the sudden activation of the unmyelinated Vagus nerve that creates this result. In addition, this disorder can be a life-long struggle or it can appear only when a person is under extreme stress.

CHAPTER 3:

The Vagus Nerve

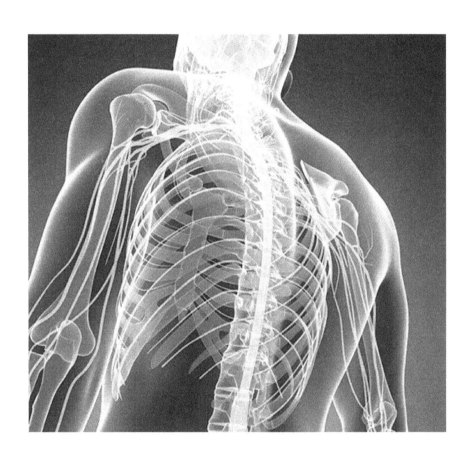

The most influential nerve that we hardly know but depend upon for our lives

Our brains contain about 100 billion neurons, or nerves, which creates a vast network of 100 trillion or so connections; this network manages every physical aspect of our bodies, from heartbeat and breathing to our senses, digestion and the functions of our liver, pancreas, kidneys, and muscles. It also manages every thought, memory and emotion we can evoke. Connecting the brain to many of the most important parts and functions of our bodies is largely the work of 12 double cranial nerves that originate in the brainstem and spread out to reach organs, muscles, and extremities. The longest, and by far the most diverse of these cranial nerves, number X in the traditional Roman numerals, is the vagus nerve; its name derives from the Latin word for the wanderer in acknowledgment of the diversity of organs and body parts it reaches.

Why should you care about a long, diverse nerve that seems to do quite well on its own, without any help or thought or acknowledgment on your part? Awake or asleep, isn't your heart beating as it should 60 times every minute; isn't your breathing going on about 14 times every minute? And aren't your kidneys doing their job filtering the waste products from your blood and forwarding them on to your bladder, and aren't your stomach and intestines doing their digestive work, and isn't your liver helping to metabolize what's been assimilated, and so on?

Yes, but there's more to this than might be apparent at first glance. While all the functions we've mentioned, and many more, are certainly under the control of the autonomic nervous system, it's component sensory and motor functions are more subject to your control than you may realize. You can have a say in how you are reacting, physically and emotionally, to the evolutionary reactions and responses that kept our early Homo Sapiens ancestors alive and ensured their inclusion in the natural selection process, but which now may be overreacting. These reactions may need to be brought down, or the reactions may be underreacting and need to be stimulated. Your vagus nerve is awaiting your introduction and acquaintance to offer you some control.

For example, we all have days when we're tense: mornings when we wake up anticipating a tough day; afternoons when the tough day actually materializes. We've had moments when a situation turns bad, when we get into an argument or disagreement, or when we experience disappointing results after we had high expectations for a positive outcome. There also stressful situations of anticipation, such as before an exam, an interview, or an important meeting. The tension is real, it's stressful, and it keeps us from being our best selves. In prehistoric times, that stress helped us run and jump out of harm's way or fight back aggressively; today, that stress can debilitate or even injure us.

Inflammation occurs as a natural and important function of the body's immune system and contributes to fighting infections. But when that system malfunctions, it can lead to continuing inflation;

that, in turn, can lead to chronic illnesses, from Type 2 diabetes and arthritis to sepsis and atherosclerosis.

Managing that tension, easing that stress, reducing that inflammation may be brought under our control, in many cases, easily with certain maneuvers and exercises we'll be covering. These exercises, which include stretches, poses, muscular contractions and releases, and a range of managed breathing actions, work because they isolate the physical cause of the tension, anxiety, and stress. The instigator is the vagus nerve, endowed by evolution to stimulate the fight or flight reactions that kept our ancestors safe when those real, existential threats were encountered. And while the vagus nerve gets our physical and emotional responses into high gear, it also can be stimulated to induce the calming effects that will bring us back down and into a state of stability and inner peace. The key is to strengthen the vagus nerve, achieving what is known as the vagal tone.

The influences of the ubiquitous vagus nerve reach from the brainstem to our hearts and lungs, our digestive system, and to other essential organs, as well as controlling our ears, nose, throat and facial muscles. It can perform all of these functions, from a smile to breath to a heartbeat, to a digestive action, because, like the other 11 cranial nerves, it's actually a double set of nerves. But unlike the others, the vagus nerve is the longest, most multitasked; no surprise that it has earned its reputation as the wanderer.

We'll begin our understanding of the vagus nerve with a look at our 12 cranial nerves and how they operate with the autonomic nervous system; a network that operates without our awareness and without our conscious help, to run our minds and bodies 24 hours a day without pause for rest or recuperation. This will lead to a look into the workings of the two nervous systems, the parasympathetic and the sympathetic, where physical and emotional responses—somatic and motor nerve functions—are generated and managed. These nervous systems react to evolutionary stimuli, pumping us up or cooling us down as required.

The most important motor functions deserve further understanding: the vagus nerve's effects on the oral cavity, the heartbeat, breathing, and digestion. We'll then move on to a newer discovery called the Polyvagal Theory, which postulates that certain physical actions, especially facial expressions, create what are called afferent influences on other parts of the body. This theory is still being tested, but there are encouraging indications of its validity.

Vagus nerve stimulation is important enough to cover in-depth, showing you certain movements, exercises, stretches and controlled breathing practices that can give you conscious control over your vagus nerve and how it influences both somatic and motor functions. The next discussion is dedicated to the electrical stimulation that medical professionals use to control the rate of the heart and arrhythmia, and in treating gastroesophageal diseases, and to control the seizures of epilepsy. We'll then move on to the more experimental forms of vagus nerve stimulation, currently being tested for slowing the progression of Alzheimer's Disease and conditions within the Asperger's Spectrum, and, finally, we'll cover the impacts of vagus nerve injuries, including digestive gastroparesis, overreactions like vasovagal syncope and other results of overstimulation.

We'll conclude our voyage alongside the wandering vagus nerve with a recap of what you can do to more effectively manage your reactions and bring them under control as you sit, lie down, walk, participate in Yoga poses and stretches, and experience the immediate effects of managed breathing.

Two Branches of the Nerve Called "Vagus"

Vagus nerve plays a small role in tasting. Carries afferent fibers from the tongue base and the epiglottis.

MOTOR FUNCTION

The vagus nerve feeds most of the muscles associated with the vagus known by the names pharynx and larynx. The muscles are involved in swallowing and vocalization.

PHARYNX

A bigger number of the muscles of the vagus nerve known as pharynx are placed in different directions by the branches of pharyngeal of the vagus nerve:

• Upper, middle and lower constrictor muscles of pharyngeal nerve

• Palatopharyngeal

• Salpingopharyngeal

LARYNX

Innervation to the muscles called intrinsic of the larynx is attained via the often recurrent laryngeal nerve also the outer branch carried by the superior laryngeal nerve.

The Recurrent laryngeal nerve:

• Thyroarytenoid

- Posterior cricoarytenoid

- Lateral cricoarytenoid

- Oblique and Transverse arytenoids

- And also Vocalis

The External laryngeal nerve:

- The Cricothyroid

- And other muscles

The Vagus Nerve: Characteristics

The vagus nerve is one of several cranial nerves or nerves that come from the brain. It consists of two parts or bundles, which link the brainstem to the rest of the body and helps control a number of bodily functions. The nerve itself, the longest nerve in your entire body, is made up of bunches of nerve cells and is part of the body's nervous system. The term vagus means "wandering", and that is precisely what the nerve does. It runs throughout the body, reaching all the way down to the colon and touching on many systems on the way down. Nearly every part of the central body is affected by the vagus nerve. All those smaller nerve endings reach out to the neck and chest, as well as the abdomen.

These nerves touch many organs, including the lungs, heart, intestines, stomach, and bladder, among others. Most people realize that the vagus nerve has an effect on things like the stomach and digestive tract, but they may not realize just how extensive it really is.

Each side of the vagus nerve has up to 100,000 nerve fibers, of which 80% are sensory. It is an essential part of the immune system, sensing when there is inflammation in the body and helping reduce it. We'll look at this in more detail in later chapters, but inflammation can cause a variety of unpleasant health conditions, and a low vagal tone is related to the increase of risk for chronic diseases like lupus and rheumatoid arthritis. Your vagus nerve helps control movement and sensory information for the heart, lungs, abdomen, and the neck, but it performs several functions in the body. However, in order to understand the functions, you need to understand something about the nervous system.

Your nervous system works in two areas, parasympathetic and sympathetic. The sympathetic part of the nervous system is responsible for boosting your heart and breathing rate, blood pressure, energy levels and how alert you are. You don't need to think about this side of things since it is all automatic.

The parasympathetic side is where the vagus nerve comes in, and it involves lowering blood pressure and heart rate, as well as alertness. It also affects the digestive system and how relaxed and calm you are. While these are the general functions of the vagus nerve, it affects more specific areas of the body. It is responsible for keeping the digestive tract working efficiently and monitoring blood pressure and sugar levels.

Nobel prize winner, Otto Loewi, discovered in 1921 that the vagus nerve affects heart rate and that the stimulation of it could actually reduce the heart rate. He realized that vagus nerve stimulation actually caused the release of a substance we now know as acetylcholine, which caused the heart to beat slower. Acetylcholine was the first neurotransmitter identified, but certainly not the last. It has also become one of the more important neurotransmitters for those of us suffering from chronic disease. Over the years, more and more scientists have studied the vagus nerve and its functions. They've discovered a remarkable number of connections and how these various connections interact with each other. When one part of the body is sick, it affects the other areas, even how we react mentally to things.

There have even been connections made between the types of food eaten and how the vagus nerve reacts. It can end up irritated and inflamed due to eating spicy food or alcohol. You can even end up with an inflamed vagus nerve when you're stressed out or anxious . . . which in turn can cause stress and anxiety. It's all connected and the vagus nerve is the center of it all. When you manage your vagus nerve and keep it in good condition, your body parts will work in unison. That's the end goal, to ensure that your entire body is working, rather than treating just one part that is causing problems. Unfortunately, that's exactly what many doctors do, treat the individual problem. However, if one of your organs is not working properly, that is going to affect more organs and it's best to look at everything as a whole.

How the Vagus Nerve Manage

The vagus nerve manages so many parts of the body that it can be devastating when something goes wrong. If there is anything that damages the nerve, such as medication, trauma, or disease, can the body heal itself? Or are you stuck with nerve damage for the rest of your life? It really all depends on how bad the damage is. Nerve damage is notorious for being slow to heal and the vagus nerve is no exception. However, scientists have tested the ability of the vagus nerve to regenerate in rats and the results have been surprising. Not only have vagus nerve techniques helped with the restoration of the central vagal parts, but they have also been shown to increase synaptic plasticity. This means that even when the brain suffers damage from damage done to the vagus nerve, it can be reversed, to a certain extent.

In tests done on rats, it took roughly 4.5 months to regenerate the central vagal nerve. That's good news for people, though it hasn't been fully tested in humans. However, studies have also shown that rebuilding the nerves in the gastrointestinal tract did not occur over the course of 45 weeks, or almost a year, which is how long the study lasted. It will definitely take time for nerves to grow back and regenerate, but the fact that it is actually possible could be exactly the hope we need.

While the central sections of the vagal nerve can be regenerated surprisingly quickly, it takes much longer to regrow the areas that branch out from it. It's important to note this because you shouldn't expect instant results from the exercises and techniques given in this book. It takes time to heal nerve damage, and that means you need to be patient and consistent if you have suffered from vagal nerve damage. Stimulation of the vagus nerve can help it grow and recover from damage. Again, it takes time, but if you are willing to put in the time and effort, you'll find that things gradually get better. As many people have discovered before you, this is not a trick. Vagus nerve stimulation really works and it can have an incredible impact on your life.

I went from barely being able to move around my house, to running marathons again. I've seen other people do even more miraculous things. And it really does seem like a miracle, but it's actually just science and your nervous system, doing their jobs. With the right stimulation, your vagus nerve will start working better than ever and becomes even more efficient. Even if you haven't suffered from any particular trauma or nerve damage, you can still expect some results from toning up your vagus nerve. It can only help you feel better and ensure that your body runs more efficiently. The amount of energy you'll have will increase and you will find that it is easier to live the lifestyle you want. There's an amazing amount of information out there if you know what to look for, yet it's still not common knowledge. I find this flabbergasting, but here you'll learn everything you need to know about how to stimulate your vagus nerve and help it recover.

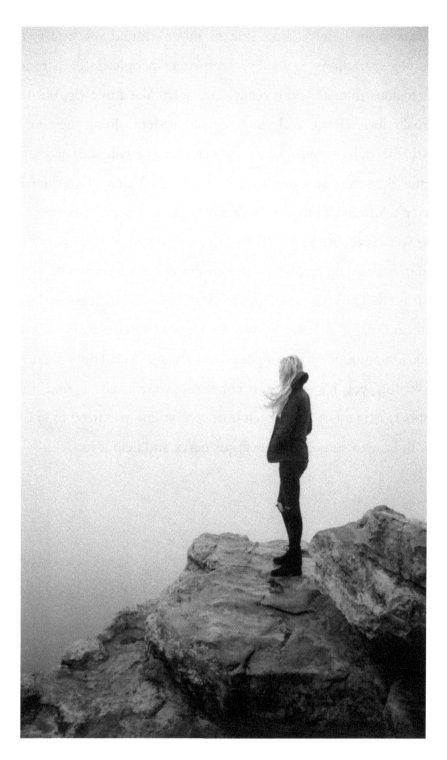

CHAPTER 4:

All the Functions of the Vagus Nerve

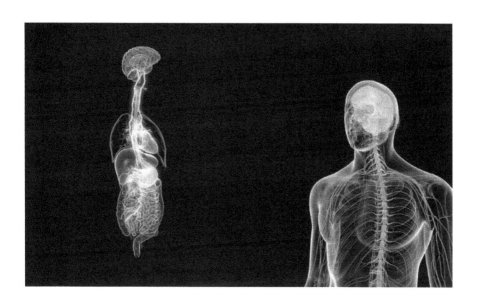

A t this point, you may wonder why I insist so much on the anatomy of the vagus nerve... The reason is very simple: it is essential to visualize inside your body the entire path carried out by such an important nerve. When you are fully aware of the presence of this nerve, it will be like having acquired a kind of superpower that will greatly facilitate its stimulation with the exercises. So now I'd like you to focus on the following description of the path of the vagus nerve, and try to visualize it first mentally, and then feel it physically. The vagus nerve emerges from the bulb through the groove of mixed nerves with a dozen of radicles and runs forward laterally to the glossopharyngeal nerve and anterior to the accessory nerve, and then it comes out of the skull through the jugular hole.

It forms the jugular ganglion and the knotty ganglion. Therefore it runs vertically in the neck. Having become independent of the glossopharyngeal and accessory nerves, it becomes part of the vascular nerve bundle of the neck, consisting of the anteromedial carotid artery and the anterior-laterally internal jugular vein.

The vagus nerve enters the chest leaving the bundle and running, right, medially to the anonymous artery and medially to the superior vena cava, to the left, laterally to the aortic arch. It moves posteriorly to the pulmonary hilum and runs, to the right, posterior to the esophagus forming the right pulmonary plexus and the posterior esophageal plexus, to the left, anteriorly to the esophagus forming the left pulmonary plexus and the anterior esophageal plexus and giving rise to the recurrent laryngeal nerve.

The anterior and posterior trunks are made up of mixed fibers, even if the posterior component is predominantly right and that of the anterior predominantly left. The vagus nerve then enters the abdomen following the course of the esophagus, passing through the diaphragmatic esophageal orifice.

In the abdomen, the two trunks run on the anterior and posterior faces of the stomach forming the anterior and posterior gastric plexuses.

The posterior branch, therefore, gives rise to the celiac branch and the celiac plexus, forming the memorable loop with the large right splanchnic nerve; the front branch gives rise to the left celiac plexus receiving the large left splanchnic. Once inside the thorax, the right and left vagus nerves to behave differently:

LEFT VAGUS NERVE

It enters the thorax between the left carotid and left subclavian arteries, and at the height of the aortic arch, it emits the left recurrent laryngeal nerve. Then it goes down and forward (becomes anterior) and passes behind the pulmonary pedicle before reaching the esophagus, where it contributes to form the esophageal plexus.

RIGHT VAGUS NERVE

It crosses in front of the right subclavian artery, and at this height, it emits the right recurrent laryngeal nerve.

Then it goes down and back (it becomes posterior) and passes behind the right pulmonary pedicle before reaching the esophagus, where it also helps to form the esophageal plexus, just like its left counterpart. Within the thorax, the vagus nerves give branches to the cardiac plexus and the pulmonary plexus.

Both vagus nerves make the last part of their journey through the thorax along with the esophagus, and next to it the abdominal cavity is introduced, crossing the diaphragm through the esophageal hiatus. Once in the abdominal cavity, the left vagus nerve is distributed through the stomach, while the right vagus nerve ends in the solar plexus from where it gives branches for the abdominal viscera (stomach, intestines, kidneys, and liver).

IT IS CONSIDERED A MIXED NERVE WITH DIFFERENT REFERENCES:

• Sensitive afference Eustachian tube, middle ear, and glossoepiglottic folds

• Parasympathetic interference Heart, bronchi, and abdominal viscera

• Ambiguous core afference. Pharyngeal style muscle (swallowing muscle)

RESEARCH AND ADDITIONAL CONSIDERATIONS ON VAGUS NERVE

With vagus nerves that have pathways to almost every organ in the body, researchers are investigating whether the stimulus is useful for other conditions.

The investigated conditions are as follows:

• Rheumatoid arthritis inflammation

• Heart failure

• Diabetes inflammation

• Unparalleled hiccups

• Abnormal heart rhythm

• Inflammation of Crohn's disease

In the case of rheumatoid arthritis, which affects 1.3 million adults in the United States, a 2016 study showed that vagus nerve stimulation could help reduce symptoms. People who did not respond to another treatment reported significant improvements, but no serious adverse side effects were observed. This was considered a breakthrough in how nerve stimulation of the vagus nerve could not only treat rheumatoid arthritis but also other inflammatory diseases, such as Crohn's disease, Parkinson's disease, and Alzheimer's disease.

The Vagus Nerve Innervates the Heart

The heartbeat is stimulated and mediated by a series of nerve clusters in the myocardium, or heart muscle. Electrical impulses are sent via the vagus nerve to the sinoatrial node (also called the sinus node), at the top of the myocardium, directly above the right atrium. The impulses then travel downward through a series of nerve clusters: atrioventricular node, the bundle of His, right and left bundle branches, and finally the Purkinje fibers. Each nerve cluster, in turn, contributes electrical impulses to simultaneously activate the right and left ventricles, causing the familiar heartbeat as blood enters the two atria, descends to the two ventricles, and is pumped out to either the aorta to reach the entire body, or the pulmonary artery, for the trip back to the lungs for reoxygenation.

The vagus nerve intervenes in lowering the heart rate because the sinoatrial node, which is known as the heart's natural pacemaker, regulates the heartbeat. The right vagus nerve innervates (fills with nerve fibers) the sinoatrial node, and uses this connection to slow the heartbeat, which usually begins at a rate of up to 100 beats per second and needs to be slowed to 60 or 70 beats. Subsequent influences of the other nerve clusters may further lower the heartbeat.

A condition known as respiratory sinus arrhythmia (RSA) is a common, normal change that happens naturally during the cycle of breathing, as the heartbeat increases during inhalation and decreases during the exhale. This effect is mediated by vagal tone, which causes rising and falling of the diaphragm to open and close the lungs, but also varying pressure within the chest cavity that influences heart rate.

The Vagus Nerve Promotes Digestion and the Functions of "Relaxation"

The link between the vagus nerve and food goes beyond its innervation in the digestive system. The intestinal flora or microbiota is a set of millions of bacteria that are responsible for helping to digest food and assist in a huge variety of functions, among which is influencing our preferences about food and visceral emotions that they drive some of our actions. This thanks to its role in the alkalinization or acidification of the intestinal environment that is perceived through the vagus nerve and interpreted as healthy and harmonic or unwanted, and can also damage the vagus nerve itself.

A correct diet allows the vagus nerve to function better, and also, our emotional and digestive health is harmonized.

It is important to avoid or reduce:

• Flours and simple carbohydrates

• Pastries and refined sweets

• Sucralose or Splenda

• Dairy animals

• Processed meats

On the other hand, the intake of the following foods should be maintained or increased:

• Green vegetables

• Papaya

• Figs

• Garlic and onion

The Vagus Nerve and Memory

It's incredible what the nervous system can do in the body and the vagus nerve is the biggest part of it. With its long-reaching pathways, it can affect nearly every part of your torso and everything in it. However, it also has a major role in the brain and the mental processes that occur there, as well as hormone release.

The vagus nerve can have an effect on your memories and thought processes. It's been linked to hormone production that stimulates the fight or flight response, feelings of happiness or contentment, and the lack of these can result in an imbalance within the brain. Anxiety, depression, and other mental health issues are all affected by the vagus nerve and whether it tells the brain to produce the necessary hormones or not.

Stimulation of the nerve has proven useful in a variety of ways. Not only can a functioning vagus nerve help prevent issues like depression or anxiety, but it can also be useful in building memories. If you need to remember things better or plan to study for an exam, it can actually help if you stimulate the vagus nerve. You'll remember better and it improves neuroplasticity or the ability to learn. In fact, it's even been shown to help with conditions like dementia and Alzheimer's. Some people use vagal stimulation as a method of improving their memory and learning over a longer period of time. It can be a very useful technique to learn.

The Vagus Nerve is an Anti-Inflammatory System

Inflammation is controlled by the vagus nerve and when it is low in tone, you will find that there is a lot more inflammation in your body. When the nerve is stimulated, it lets the immune system know that it should calm down. The result is less chronic inflammation and better health. Your immune system can malfunction just like everything else in the body, but when it does, it has widespread effects. Chronic inflammation will cause poor health and can even result in death if it gets bad enough. That's right, your own body can actually kill you if the inflammation gets out of control. This is why people die from autoimmune diseases.

It's obviously best to prevent mistaken immune system responses, but the current method is to dose people up with medications that lower the immune system. These are the same drugs used to treat cancer and they have their own side effects. It's also not a good idea to restrict your immune system for long periods of time, as this can leave you open to a lot of other diseases and will limit your lifestyle.

It's far better to aim for natural methods of reducing inflammation. Eating a healthy diet and eliminating sugar and processed foods from your diet is a good start, but frequent stimulation of the vagus nerve is also useful. It will help your body lower the inflammation and prevent the creation of more white blood cells, which can be an issue when there are too many of them.

CHAPTER 5:

Vagus Nerve Dysfunction

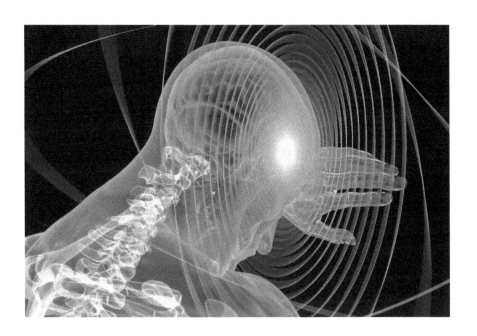

Damage To The Vagus Nerve

The abuse of alcohol can lead to a condition called alcoholic neuropathy; large, frequent quantities of alcohol can create toxic damage to the key components of the autonomic nervous system, including the vagus nerve. Dramatically reduced consumption can often reverse these damaging effects.

Infections to the upper respiratory system can lead to post-viral vagal neuropathy, a condition caused by prolonged coughing, nasal congestion, and nasal discharge. Symptoms include chronic coughing, difficulty swallowing, and speaking difficulties. Another cause of vagus nerve damage can occur during surgery to repair and cure ulcers and gastric acid reflux damage. Another form of digestion-related damage is digestive gastroparesis.

Digestive Gastroparesis

When the vagus nerve is damaged or malfunctioning, it can affect the digestive system; a condition known as digestive gastroparesis occurs when the muscles in the stomach are unable to process and move food forward to the small intestine. Peristalsis, the contracts and expansions that advance the food do not function effectively.

The causes of digestive gastroparesis are often unknown but in addition to a damaged vagus nerve (caused by surgery, for example), it may be caused by uncontrolled diabetes, narcotics and medications, Parkinson's disease, multiple sclerosis, and in very rare cases, certain connective tissue disorders.

Symptoms range from heartburn and GERD (acid reflux complications), bloating, loss of appetite and feeling full prematurely, and nausea. Undigested food that remains in the stomach may ferment and be susceptible to bacterial infection.

Results of Overstimulation: Vasovagal Syncope

Overstimulation of the vagus nerve by non-electrical stimuli can cause dizziness, disorientation, and fainting. Fainting is caused by a condition called vasovagal syncope; in stressful or traumatic situations, the heartbeat and blood pressure levels go up, and to compensate, the blood supply to the brain is reduced by the vagus nerve becoming overexcited. This can occur when a person experiences stress. Common examples of vasovagal syncope causing fainting are the sight of blood, seeing an injured person, receiving an injection or watching someone else be injected. In response to these stress-inducing events, the overstimulated vagus nerve causes the heart rate to drop and blood pressure to drop.

In many situations of the onset of vagal overstimulation, the person experiences lightheadedness, and by sitting or lying down, the overstimulation passes, and there are no further effects. But in the extreme, fainting or unconsciousness can occur:

A woman in California reported that she stood up suddenly to walk into the kitchen. She picked up a jar to gather leftovers, and the next thing she knew was that her husband was trying to arouse her; she had fainted and fell to the floor. Apparently, her abrupt standing up and walking briskly caused a rise in heart rate and blood pressure, overstimulating the vagus nerve, triggering vasovagal syncope.

The intensity of exercise can induce vagal overstimulation, especially among individuals who are not well-conditioned and overdo the running or elliptical or Stairmaster challenges in their fitness center. The heart is being asked to beat more rapidly to supply more oxygen, the lungs are breathing harder and faster, and the result can be an overstimulated vagus nerve that wants to shut things down; heart rate slows, blood pressure drops and passing out becomes a very real option for the body. A similar effect can occur among conditioned athletes who start out too fast, not allowing their heart and respiratory system sufficient time to warm up.

Dysfunctional Breathing

The Vagus nerve has the primary function of offering stimulation to the vocal chord's muscles. If your vagus nerve has any sort of damage or dysfunction, there is a probability that these muscles will be damaged as well. This then interferes with both your breathing ability and your voice. Other muscles are supported by the function of the Vagus nerve as well. You may feel like your electrolytes are low, such as your potassium or magnesium levels, which cause muscle cramps, but those cramps may also be caused by damage to your Vagus nerve.

Poor circulation: In some people, poor circulation is an unpleasant sign of a low vagal tone. When your hands and feet tend to get cold, but the rest of the body is fine, it may be caused by a lack of circulation. The blood just isn't reaching as far as it should. Since the vagus nerve is responsible for your heart rate, it is a big part of this disease and needs to be considered when dealing with low circulation.

Pulmonary disease: Your lungs are also controlled by the vagus nerve and it stimulates regular breathing. Poor lung health, COPD, and other types of pulmonary disease can all affect the vagal tone in the body.

Dysfunctional Microbiome

Now it is clear why it is so important. Many symptoms of different organs may be related to it. One of the most interesting roles of the vagus nerve is that it basically monitors the microbiome (colonies of bacteria, viruses and other germs that live in our gut) and triggers an answer to regulate inflammation based on whether it detects pathogens against non-pathogens organisms.

In this way, the gut microbiome can have a positive effect on mood and stress levels and reduce overall inflammation and therefore, the pain caused by it.

For example, given the importance of the vagus nerve in the intestine, when it is not functioning properly it becomes a cause of digestive disorders such as dyspepsia, gastroparesis, esophageal reflux, ulcerative colitis, anorexia, and bulimia, to name a few.

The vagus nerve is an important part of the parasympathetic nervous system, in addition to affecting mental health; it affects digestive function and breathing, and heart rate. In this book, you will explore the wonders and secrets of the vagus nerve and learn step-by-step exercises to stimulate and enhance its functions. You will enjoy a quick relief from your symptoms and become much stronger and healthy.

Chronic Inflammation and Immune Activation

Nearly every autoimmune disease is caused by inflammation in the body. In fact, a great number of diseases, in general, are due to inflammation in the tissues. It is a big problem and one that pills can't really fix, though anti-inflammatories will lower it somewhat.

Inflammation has been linked to some of the most deadly diseases today, including diabetes, cancer, stroke, heart disease, and others. It has also been connected to autism and mental health issues, as well as a number of other brain diseases. Inflammation can kill you, but it's not entirely bad.

A study done by Dr. Harold A. Silverman at the Laboratory for Biomedical Science at the Feinstein Institute for Medical Research showed some interesting connections between inflammation and the vagus nerve. It showed that if the vagus nerve has a low tone, then the body is at higher risk for increased and chronic inflammation. This prolonged inflammation could cause issues like rheumatoid arthritis and other conditions associated with long-term inflammation in the body.

Dysfunctional Liver Function

It may develop as a chronic subclinical and cellular disturbance. Also can go on to be life-threatening, also said to be a hepatic failure with more organ system compromise. The vagus nerve plays a series of vital roles in the digestive system, helping to control the continuing process of food descending from the mouth, passing the epiglottis, entering the esophagus, passing the esophageal sphincter, entering the stomach where the vagus nerve ensures food is prepared for assimilation and pushed forward into the small intestine, where assimilation actually occurs. It further ensures the food continues to be digested as it continues into the large intestine and the traverse portion of the colon. Vagal fibers also extend into the liver and pancreas.

As it descends, the vagus nerve reaches and influences all components of the digestive system. Together these connections form the esophageal plexus. In this series of connections, the vagus nerve plays a diversity of roles in controlling the digestive process. One notable effect is the mediation of peristalsis, the automatic contractions and expansions that move food from the stomach into the small intestine. When this process is malfunctioning, it can lead to a condition called gastroparesis, in which the contractions fail to move food through the stomach, causing loss of appetite, pain, nausea, and malnutrition.

The vagus nerve plays a critical health maintenance role in the gastroesophageal system by preventing acid reflux, which can lead to gastroesophageal reflux disease (GERD). It facilitates blocking gastric hydrochloric acid (HCL) from entering the esophagus by managing the pressure of the esophageal sphincter (which closes the opening at the top of the stomach).

Chronic Stress

Your body's levels of stress hormones are regulated by the autonomic nervous system (SNA). SNA has two components that balance each other: the sympathetic nervous system (SNS) and the parasympathetic nervous system (SPS).

SNS increases nervous system activity. It helps manage what we perceive as an emergency and is responsible for responding to getaways.

SPS reduces nervous system activity and keeps you calm. Slowing down, your heart rate promotes relaxation, rest, sleep, and drowsiness. This slows breathing, contracts the pupils of the eyes, and increases saliva production in the mouth, and as we know it is largely controlled by the vagus nerve

This nervous system uses acetylcholine, a neurotransmitter. If the brain cannot communicate with the diaphragm through the release of acetylcholine from the vagus nerve (for example, if it is affected by botulinum toxin), it stops breathing and dies.

Acetylcholine is involved in learning and memory. It also calms and relaxes you. Used by the vagus nerve to send peace and relaxation messages throughout the body. New research has discovered that acetylcholine acts as an important brake on inflammation in the body. In other words, by stimulating the vagus nerve, it not only relaxes but also sends acetylcholine throughout the body by extinguishing the inflammation fire associated with the negative effects of stress.

Acute stress disorders, like PTSD, occur in response to traumatic events and have similar symptoms. However, symptoms occur from 3 days to 1 month after the event.

People with acute stress disorders can rejuvenate trauma, feel flashbacks and nightmares, get paralyzed, and leave themselves.

These symptoms can cause great distress and cause problems in daily life. About half of people with acute stress disorder have PTSD.

An estimated 13-21% of car accident survivors develop acute stress disorder, and 20-50% of survivors of assault, rape, or mass shooting develop it.

Psychotherapy, including cognitive-behavioral therapy, helps control symptoms and prevents them from getting worse and becoming PTSD. Drugs such as SSRI antidepressants can help relieve symptoms.

Vasovagal Syncope and Valsalva Maneuver

Pharmaceutical interventions and agents will be wont to influence the cranial nerve tone of the guts thereby speed it down a number of them area unit beta-blockers, muscarinic agents, digitalis area unit simply many to be mentioned.

In innate heart defects like patent duteous arteriosus, there may be associate degree irritation to the cranial nerve, and this could end in speech disorder, which is hoarseness of the voice.

Excessive activation of the cranial nerve throughout stress, that could be a parasympathetic response, may end up in eliciting a stronger sympathetic counter-reaction, which successively will cause vasovagal syncope that is an explosive reduction inflow.

The agent during this case will be:

1. Standing for a protracted time

2. Straining once attempting to possess a BM

3. Fear of close hurt

4. Exposure to extreme heat

Vasovagal syncope happens in ladies and youngsters and may result in loss of bladder management below extreme worry. Moreover, throughout emotional stress, an arterial massage will with success compress the arteria sinus and result in a high pressure, a sequel to this; the cranial nerve can be got to increase its activities, so the sino-atrial node of the guts, also because the heart muscle can reduce their contraction. Thanks to the decrease in the contraction of the guts, syncope may occur.

Although lesions to the cranial nerve area unit rare, a lesion to the tubular cavity branches of the cranial nerve may end up in a problem in swallowing, (dysphagia), and thanks to the weakness of the muscles of the tubular cavity being innervated by the cranial nerve. The cranial nerve is additionally sensory to the cavity and cavum.

Research has additionally unconcealed the chance of ladies having the ability to expertise consummation, whereas having sustained medulla spinal injury. The cranial nerve is that the principal agent is that the stimulation of orgasms within the context which may go from the womb and cervix to the brain.

Valsalva Maneuver could be a technique that has been followed in medication and additionally in a way of life. It helps increase the tone of the cranial nerve and additionally at the same time increasing the tone within the throat, sinuses, and ears. It's a vital technique for ventilator different, and other people experiencing a variable degree of supraventricular tachycardia. Valsalva maneuver will increase the pressures within the nasal sinuses aboard the thoracic cavity.

The elevated chest pressure ends up in a stimulation of the cranial nerve, thereby increasing the cranial nerve tone; it then results in a sequence of physiological events that helps the body. The increment within the cranial nerve tone reduces the speed of the physical phenomenon of internal organ electrical impulses through the AV node. This reduction in the physical phenomenon helps terminate some varieties of supraventricular tachycardia (AV-nodal re-entrant tachycardia and atrioventricular re-entrant tachycardia). This suggests that folks who expertise continual episodes on these forms of Supraventricular tachycardia will greatly cut back the speed of the heart disease through the Valsalva maneuver.

Lack of Social Interaction

Positive social interactions have been shown to cause the activation of the vagus nerve, which means you need that interaction with other people. Even introverts can benefit from talking to someone else, sharing a meal, or engaging in activity that is shared with another person, or multiple people. However, these interactions must remain positive since negative interactions and relationships can actually lower vagal tone.

When interacting with someone else, there are a few ways to increase the vagal tone benefits for both of you. First, establish a meaningful, connected relationship with the other person. This will help both of you. Making eye contact and physical connection can also be beneficial. Hugs are a terrific way to stimulate the vagus nerve, thanks to both physical pressure and positive associations.

You've probably noticed that when you get a hug from someone, it just feels really good. Some people are better huggers than others, but the connection strengthens with hugs and physical contact, making it more likely that you'll continue the relationship and view it in a positive light. All of this is good for your vagal tone and should be pursued whenever possible.

Conclusion

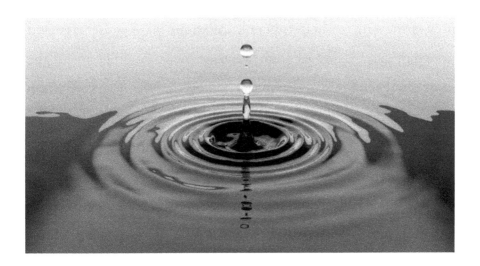

Congratulations on making it through to the end of this journey on the vagus nerve, a scientific guide to understand how the vagus nerve determines psychological and emotional states such as anxiety, depression, migraines, back pain, and with simple exercises to improve your life.

Hopefully, it was full of information and offered tools that you need to help you achieve your goals.

The next step in your journey to understand your body and your Vagus nerve is to give stimulation techniques a shot. It is time to decide what exercises you want to try and put them into action. It is not enough to just read about all the functions of the Vagus nerve and how it can be stimulated or balanced. It is now time to apply your knowledge and change your life. And not only that, now is the time to help others learn about the Vagus nerve and how they can balance or stimulate their own. Possibly one of the most interesting outcomes of this book is that the final suggestion is to create connections with others in a genuine and wholehearted manner. And the more you build these connections the better you support their Vagus nerve stimulation, as well as your own. You can help others, ultimately help yourself, and create a more relaxed, peaceful, and balanced lifestyle. So if you are struggling with a technique outlined in this book and are unsure where to start, it is time to create these loving and kind relationships. It is time to develop deep connections with others and build a positive environment around yourself and others. This is one of the most effective methods for not only creating a great environment but also support the function of your Vagus nerve.

Thank you for reading and please take good care of your body.

CPSIA information can be obtained
at www.ICGtesting.com
Printed in the USA
BVHW061406250321
603170BV00020B/923